# CONTROL AND PREVENTION OF INFECTIOUS DISEASES

Simple Guide on Infection Treatment, Strategies for Managing and Stopping Infectious Disease, Proactive Approaches and Effective Solutions

**GEORGE LEO**

Copyright © 2024 George Leo

All rights reserved.

# DEDICATION

To the countless individuals and families who have faced the trials of infectious diseases with courage and resilience, and to the healthcare workers who tirelessly fight on the front lines. This book is dedicated to the scientists and public health professionals whose unwavering commitment brings us closer to a healthier world. May their efforts inspire hope and bring about a future free from the shadow of infectious diseases.

# TABLE OF CONTENTS

DEDICATION ..................................................................................... iii
TABLE OF CONTENTS ..................................................................... v
ACKNOWLEDGMENTS ..................................................................... i
INTRODUCTION ............................................................................... ii
CHAPTER 1 ........................................................................................ 1
ROUTES OF INFECTION ................................................................. 1
CHAPTER 2 ........................................................................................ 4
SOURCES OF HEALTHCARE ASSOCIATED INFECTION ............ 4
CHAPTER 3 ........................................................................................ 5
TYPES OF NOSOCOMIAL INFECTIONS ....................................... 5
CHAPTER 4 ........................................................................................ 8
CLASSIFICATION OF WOUNDS .................................................... 8
CHAPTER 5 ...................................................................................... 10
BASICS ISSUES OF INFECTION CONTROL ............................... 10
CHAPTER 6 ...................................................................................... 14
PRINCIPLES OF INFECTION CONTROL .................................... 14
CHAPTER 7 ...................................................................................... 20
LABORATORY INVESTIGATIONS OF HAIs .............................. 20
CHAPTER 8 ...................................................................................... 22
INFECTION CONTROL COMMITTEE ......................................... 22
CHAPTER 9 ...................................................................................... 25
INFECTION PREVENTION AND CONTROL NURSE ................ 25
CHAPTER 10 .................................................................................... 28
INFECTION AFTER SURGERY ..................................................... 28
CHAPTER 11 .................................................................................... 33

George Leo

| | |
|---|---|
| KITCHEN AND FOOD SAFETY | 33 |
| CHAPTER 12 | 36 |
| OUT BREAK CONTROL | 36 |
| CHAPTER 13 | 42 |
| GLOBAL HEALTH SECURITY | 42 |
| CONCLUSION | 51 |

# ACKNOWLEDGMENTS

Creating Control and Prevention of Infectious Diseases has been a profound and humbling experience. I am deeply grateful to the dedicated healthcare professionals who risk their lives daily to protect us. Your courage and kindness are at the core of this work.

To the scientists and researchers whose tireless efforts have expanded our understanding of infectious diseases, thank you. Your continuous quest for knowledge and innovation fills us with hope for a healthier future.

I am grateful to my family and friends for their wonderful support and encouragement. Your steady belief in me has been a wellspring of strength throughout this journey. During the most challenging moments, your belief in this project kept me moving forward.

Finally, to all those affected by infectious diseases, your strength and resilience are an inspiration. This book is for you, and I hope it contributes to a world where these diseases are no longer a threat.

# INTRODUCTION

Infection Control and Prevention for Health Care Providers and individual that values their health is a clear and concise guide to preventing occupational exposure hazards and communicable and infectious diseases. The hospital environment is a place where many individuals, often with weakened immune systems, are gathered due to illness. Therefore measures must be put in place to prevent these patients from acquiring other infections or contacting more diseases.

# CHAPTER 1

# ROUTES OF INFECTION

**Infection can be acquired either from:**

- Endogenous route- where the source is from the microorganisms is from the patient's own micro-flora e.g. from the gut due to break in intestinal barriers caused by the chemotherapy in cancer patients.
- Exogenous route: This is when microorganisms originate from external sources outside the body e.g. from contaminated hands of healthcare workers, as well as from items, equipment, or the surrounding environment.
- It should be noted that every exposure to microorganisms does not necessarily lead to infection.
- The risk of infection is a constant concern in healthcare settings.

## Health care associated infection includes:

- Not existing or developing at the time of admission
- These are infections that arise more than 48 hours after a patient has been admitted.
- These are infections acquired in the hospital but that become apparent only after the patient has been discharged from the healthcare facility.
- Occupational infections among health care staff.

## Definition

- Nosocomial infections (NI) or hospital acquired infections or Health care associated infections (HAI) are those infections which are acquired a result of treatment in a health care facility but are secondary to the patient's original condition.
- Health Care Associated Infections are also defined as infections acquired during the delivery of health care while receiving treatment from or visiting a health facility.

- Infections are considered nosocomial if they appear **48hours or more** after hospital admission or within **30 days after discharge.**

# CHAPTER 2

# SOURCES OF HEALTHCARE ASSOCIATED INFECTION

- Staff and attendants' hands (through the use of buckets and bowls)
- Hand washing solid soap and communal towels
- No hand washing
- Assisted ventilation equipment.
- Suction and drainage bottles.
- I.V. lines – central and peripheral
- Urinary catheters- especially metal catheters.
- Wounds and wound dressings
- Disinfectant containers
- Dressing trolleys
- Bed frames.

## MICROBIAL AGENT
Developing of clinical disease depends on:

1. Organism's virulence- the more the virulence the higher the chances of developing a disease.

2. Infective dose: The higher the dose of the infectious agent, the greater the likelihood of infection.

3. Patient resistance- patients with weak or impaired host resistance are more prone to developing an infection.

**Bacteria are the most common pathogens.**

1. Commensal bacteria: typically present in the normal flora of healthy individuals, prevent pathogenic bacterial colonization e.g. skin, colon, vagina. They are the most commonly implicated.

2. Pathogenic bacteria possess significant virulence and can cause infections such as:

- Anaerobic gram positive rods e.g. Clostridium perfringes causing gas gangrene, Bacillus spp. Clostridium difficile
- Gram positive bacteria: Staphylococcus aureus found on skin & nose; Coagulase – negative staphylococci.
- Beta hemolytic Streptococcus spp. – S. agalactiae, S. progenies.

- Gram-negative bacteria, such as E. coli, Proteus spp., *Klebsiella* spp., Pseudomonas spp., and Acinetobacter baumannii.
- Legionella species.

**Other organisms that can be implicated include:**

**3. Viruses:** HIV, HBV, HCV can be also be transmitted through blood & blood products (transfusion, injections, dialysis) Respiratory Syncytial virus, Rota virus, Ebola virus, Influenza virus, Para influenza virus, Herpes simplex viruses.

**4. Parasites:** e.g. Giardia lamblia is easily transmitted between adults or children; Scabies an ectoparasite cause bSyarcoptes scabiei causing outbreak.

**5. Fungi**: Aspergillus sp . Spores can contaminate the environment affecting immunocompromised Patients. Others includeC: ryptococcus neoformans.

**Patient Susceptibility**

- Age: Infants and elderly individuals have reduced resistance to infections.
- Immune status: Patients with chronic conditions such as malignancy, leukemia, diabetes mellitus, renal failure, or AIDS have heightened susceptibility to

infections.

- Immunosuppressive drugs or irradiation: Chemotherapy for cancer, steroids, radiotherapy.

Environmental Factors

Poor ventilation.

Crowded conditions within hospital.

Frequent transfers of patients between units.

Use of contaminate objects, devices and materials.

The highest rate of infection occurred in the burns ICU, the Special Care Baby Unit (S.C.B.U) and the pediatrics ICU.

# CHAPTER 3

# TYPES OF NOSOCOMIAL INFECTIONS

**1. Bloodstream and catheter infection:** Often indicated by inflammation, lymphangitis, or purulent discharge at the insertion site. There may be fever or rigor and at least one positive blood culture.

**2. Surgical site infections:** Any purulent discharge, abscesses, spreading cellulitis at the surgical site month after the surgery.

**3. Urinary tract infection:** Positive urine culture ( 1 or 2 species) in 100000 bacteria/ml, with or without clinical symptoms.

**4. Respiratory or ventilator associated HA infection:** Respiratory symptoms with at least 2 signs which include cough, purulent sputum, new infiltrate on chest appearing during hospitalization.

## Blood Stream Infection (BSIs)

- Could be primary or secondary from other foci.

It can happen if the catheter has been in place for:

- Less than 5days: peripheral line
- 5 – 10days Central Venous Catheter (Jugular vein)
- 5 – 28days: Central Venous Catheter (Subclavian)
- >28days – Hickmann's catheter (Tunneled lines)

## CARE OF BLOOD STREAM INFECTIONS

- . Proper skin care before insertion- use disinfectants like 70% alcohol, povidone iodine.

- Insertion site is the usual focus of infection in the 1st 2weeks so closely monitor this place.

- The hub after 2 weeks becomes the next focus of infection.

- Material of catheter used – Teflon, Polyurethane or silicon better

- Golden rule: remove as soon as possible; don't keep it longer than necessary.

## PREVENTION OF CLABSI

Subclavian vein best, not jugular, never use femoral vein.

Frequency of dressing change is important.

Adherence to aseptic techniques is critical.

Use of topical antibiotic is not advisable.

# CHAPTER 4

# CLASSIFICATION OF WOUNDS

**Class I – Clean wounds:** No entry into the RS, GIT or UGS

**Class II – Clean contaminated:** The RS, UGS, GIT are entered into but under controlled conditions and without contamination.

**Class III – Contaminated:** These are usually accidental wounds/ breaks in sterile technique.

**Class IV** – Dirty Infected wounds with retained devitalized tissue $\pm$ perforated viscera $\pm$ clinical condition.

## SOURCES OF WOUND INFECTION
- Endogenous source- 80 – 90% of cases are from the micro flora of the patient.

- Exogenous source -5 – 15% of most wound

infections are from external sources e.g. from other patients' wounds or from contaminated dressing materials.

- The type of wound infection is predicted by number of organisms (especially bacteria) entering the wound, the type of microorganism, the virulence of the organism and the immunity of the host.

- For instance, the risk is heightened if the site is contaminated with over 100,000 organisms per gram of tissue.

- .Pre- operative hospitalization also increases the risk of acquiring SSI.

# CHAPTER 5

# BASICS ISSUES OF INFECTION CONTROL

Prevention of nosocomial infection is the responsibility of ALL individuals involved in the services provided by healthcare setting.

To practice good asepsis, one should always be able to separate and differentiate between:

**What is dirty?**

**What is clean?**

**What is sterile?**

Hospital policies and procedures must be applied to prevent spread of infection in hospital.

## PRECAUTION IN THE PREVENTION OF INFECTION

There are two type of precaution taken in the health

care setting to prevent infection:

- Transmission based or additional precaution.
- Standard precautions

**Standard precautions are guidelines**

Designed to create a physical, mechanical, or chemical barrier between microorganisms and a person to prevent the spread of infection (i.e the barrier helps to interrupt the disease transmission cycle).

## DEFINITION OF STANDARD PRECAUTIONS

- Standard precautions are precautions that are designed to reduce the risk of transmission of microorganisms from both recognized and unrecognized sources of infection in healthcare settings, and apply to all individuals, irrespective of their medical condition or suspected infectious condition.

- Standard precautions are applicable to every patient, irrespective of their specific diagnosis.

## EXAMPLES OF STANDARD PRECAUTIONS

- Physical: Personal protective equipment (PPE) (gloves, face masks, goggles, gowns, plastic or rubber aprons, and drapes).

- Mechanical: by boiling or steaming and sterilization by autoclaving or dry heat ovens.

- Chemical: Substances such as alcohol-based antiseptics and potent disinfectants like chlorine and glutaraldehyde.

## TRANSMISSION OR ADDITIONAL BASED PRECAUTIONS

Transmission based precautions are guidelines designed to reduce risk of transmitting infections that are spread by organisms with known mode of transmission which could be by airborne, droplet, or contact routes between hospitalized patients, and health providers.

## TRANSMISSION BASED PRECAUTION INCLUDES:

- Patient placement

- Patient transport

- Respiratory protection

- Gloving

- Hand hygiene

## George Leo

- Cough etiquette

- After-patient contact

- Patient care equipment

- Donning, removal and care of PPE

.

# CHAPTER 6

# PRINCIPLES OF INFECTION CONTROL

The basis of infection control practices is the use of practices or procedures that prevents or reduce the likelihood of infection being transmitted from a source (e.g. person, contaminated body fluids, equipment and environment) to another susceptible individual. These practices include:

1. **Hand washing:** Washing of hands with or without the use of alcohol rubs by ALL medical personnel before each patient contact is a single way that has been shown to help minimize the spread of infections within the hospital.

2. **Personal Protective Equipment:** lab\ ward coats, aprons; face masks; goggles; caps; boots and hand gloves. Hand gloves are worn to protect the health care provider from blood borne pathogens and

to also reduce the likelihood that the microorganisms in the provider's hands can be transmitted to the patient during invasive procedures. They must be changed between patients contact

**3. Cleaning, Disinfection, and Sterilization:** Cleaning involves physically removing organic material or soil from surfaces or objects.

Commonly cleaned items include the floor and windows.

**4. Management of waste:** The World Health Organization (WHO) defines healthcare waste as the complete waste stream generated by a healthcare or research facility, encompassing both potentially hazardous (risk) waste and non-hazardous (non-risk) waste materials.

- Waste must be made safe before disposal.
- This can be done through autoclaving, disinfection, or incineration of sharps.
- All health care waste should be packed in color coded bags.

**5. Management of linen:** Cleaning, disinfection and sterilization of patient's supplies should be performed in the central sterile services department (CSSD All items should be meticulously cleaned prior to sterilization. Presoaking in disinfectant is ineffective and should be discouraged. Soiled linens should be kept in white or clear bag before sending to CSSD.

**6. Management of blood spillage:** Blood is a medium that can contain potentially infectious and highly virulent agent. Blood spills should be cleaned using a 1:10 dilution of hypochlorite solution. This dilution should be replaced after 24hours because they decay rapidly once diluted.

**7. Management of inoculation and contamination accidents:** Needle stick injuries, surgical accidents and other forms of accidents should be quickly managed to prevent disease establishment.

## Essential Measures for Infection Prevention in Healthcare Settings

Standard Precautions stand as the cornerstone of infection prevention protocols in healthcare environments. These guidelines, rooted in evidence-based practices, are paramount for safeguarding the health of both patients and healthcare workers, irrespective of the infectious status of individuals.

**8. Hand Hygiene:** The simple act of hand hygiene

serves as a fundamental barrier against the transmission of pathogens. Regular and thorough hand washing, alongside the use of alcohol-based hand rubs, is imperative for maintaining cleanliness and preventing infection spread.

**Respiratory Hygiene (Cough Etiquette):** To curb the dissemination of respiratory infections, practicing respiratory hygiene and cough etiquette is indispensable. This entails covering one's mouth and nose when coughing or sneezing, disposing of used tissues promptly, and maintaining meticulous hand hygiene thereafter.

**Personal Protective Equipment (PPE):** Selecting appropriate PPE is crucial to mitigate the risk of contamination. Factors such as the nature of anticipated exposure, durability of the equipment, and proper fit must be considered to ensure effective protection against blood borne pathogens and bodily fluids.

**Aseptic Technique:** Maintaining aseptic conditions during medical procedures is paramount to prevent infections. Different levels of aseptic technique, ranging from standard to surgical asepsis, dictate the extent of precautions required to minimize contamination risks.

## Needle-stick and Sharps Injury Prevention:

Implementing safe injection practices is imperative to prevent needle-stick injuries and subsequent transmission of blood borne pathogens. Adhering to standard precautions and aseptic techniques forms the foundation of safe injection practices.

**Cleaning and Disinfection:** Thorough reprocessing of reusable medical equipment between patient uses is essential to prevent cross-contamination. Using the right rules for cleaning, killing germs, and making things germ-free makes medical tools safe and works well.

**Waste Disposal:** Effective waste management is vital for minimizing infection transmission risks. Proper containment and disposal of waste materials in designated areas help prevent the spread of infectious agents within healthcare facilities.

# George Leo

Finally, sticking to safety steps like washing hands and wearing protective gear is super important in hospitals to stop germs from spreading. By implementing these evidence-based measures consistently, healthcare facilities can uphold a safe and hygienic environment for both patients and healthcare personnel.

# CHAPTER 7

# LABORATORY INVESTIGATIONS OF HAIs

**Microscopy:** Gram stain of samples taken from suspected sites of infection.

**Bloodstream culture:** Samples from the I.V Line and peripheral vein assessments are conducted to assist in the differential diagnosis of the line.

**Fungal cultures:** Culture media include Saboraud's agar, Cornmeal agar. Indian ink stain. KOH wet mount.

**Immunofluorescence test for influenza, Respiratory syncytial virus transmitted by contact; and Others:** Special imaging techniques e.g. Ultrasonography, CT scans, and MRI can be helpful in assessing difficult-to-detect infections, such as those caused by Pneumocystis jirovecii.

## PREVENTION OF HCAIS

- The primary focus of preventive efforts should be in hospitals and other healthcare facilities.
- Risk prevention for patients and staff is a collective responsibility within the facility and must be endorsed by senior administration.

An annual work plan should be developed to evaluate and promote good healthcare practices, appropriate isolation, sterilization, staff training, and epidemiological surveillance.

# CHAPTER 8

# INFECTION CONTROL COMMITTEE

An Infection Control Committee serves as a platform for multidisciplinary input, cooperation, and information sharing. This committee should include broad representation from relevant programs, such as management, physicians, other healthcare workers, clinical microbiology, pharmacy, central supply, maintenance, housekeeping, and training services. It should report directly to either administration or medical staff to ensure the program's visibility and effectiveness.

In emergencies, such as an outbreak, the committee must be able to convene promptly.

**The committee has the following tasks:**

To evaluate and authorize an annual plan of activities focused on surveillance and prevention efforts.

- To assess epidemiological surveillance data and

pinpoint areas for intervention.

• To evaluate and advocate for enhanced practices across all levels of the healthcare facility.

• To guarantee adequate staff training in infection control and safety measures.

• To assess risks linked with new technologies and monitor infectious risks associated with new devices and products before their approval for use.

• To assess and participate in epidemic investigations.

• To communicate and cooperate with other committees of the hospital with common interests such as Pharmacy and Therapeutics or Antimicrobial Use Committee, Biosafety or Health and Safety, and Blood Transfusion Committee.

## INFECTION CONTROL TEAM

The infection control team or individual is tasked with overseeing the day-to-day operations of infection control.

For preparing the yearly work plan for review by the infection control committee and administration. In some countries, these professionals are part of specialized teams serving a single hospital or a network of healthcare facilities. They might be administratively integrated into another unit. For example, a microbiology laboratory, medical or nursing administration, or public health services may be involved. The ideal structure will differ based on the type, requirements, and resources of the facility.

# CHAPTER 9

# INFECTION PREVENTION AND CONTROL NURSE

An Infection Prevention and Control (IPC) nurse is a registered nurse with specialized academic education and practical training in infection control.

The IPC nurse should possess effective communication skills to engage with staff of all levels, negotiate and implement changes, and influence practices positively.

FUNCTIONS OF THE IPC NURSE

• Serves as a specialist advisor and take a leading day-to-day role in the effective function of the IPC team.

• He or She must be an active member of the hospital IPC committee.

• Should assist the hospital IPC committee to draw up annual plans and policies.

Offers specialized nursing expertise in the surveillance, prevention, monitoring, and management of Healthcare-Associated Infections (HAIs).

• Identifies, investigates, and promptly addresses all hazardous practices and procedures related to Infection Prevention and Control (IPC).

• Provides guidance to contracting departments and participates in preparing documents related to service specifications and quality standards.

• Ongoing contribution to the development and implementation of the IPC policies and procedures, participating in the audit and develops monitoring tools related to IPC and infectious diseases.

Presentation of educational program and membership of relevant committees where IPC input is required.

## EFFECT OF REDUCTION IN HEALTHCARE ASSOCIATED INFECTIONS

- Reduced length of stay
- Fewer medication errors
- Lower rates of ventilator-associated pneumonia
- Lower rates of bloodstream infection
- Fewer decubitus ulcers (Bed sores)
- Higher employee morale
- Lower staff burnout
- Less absenteeism.

# CHAPTER 10

# INFECTION AFTER SURGERY

A Surgical Site Infection (SSI) develops when pathogens proliferate at the site of a surgical incision, resulting in an infection. While urinary tract infections and respiratory infections can occur following any surgery, SSIs are specific to surgeries that require an incision. Surgical site infections (SSIs) are relatively common, occurring in 2-6% of surgeries that involve incisions. Rates of infection differ consistent with the type of surgery. Up to Six Hundred Thousand (600,000) surgical site infections (SSIs) occur yearly in the United States. Most SSIs are staph infections. The major causes of are germs that goes into your body during or after surgery activities. In severe cases, surgical site infections (SSIs) can lead to complications like sepsis, a bloodstream infection that may result in organ failure.

An SSI is defined as an infection that develops at the site of a surgical wound within 30 days of the incision Symptoms of a Surgical Site Infection (SSI) following surgery include:

- A Surgical Site Infection (SSI) that solely impacts the superficial layers of skin surrounding the stitches is referred to as a superficial infection.
- Bacteria from your skin, the air, a surgeon's hands, and other surfaces in the hospital can be transferred into your wound around the time of your surgical procedure. As your immune system focuses on recovery from surgery, these germs can multiply at the site of the infection.

Such infections are typically painful but often respond positively to antibiotic treatment. Occasionally, your doctor may need to surgically reopen a portion of your incision to facilitate drainage.

## MUSCLE AND TISSUE WOUND INFECTION AFTER SURGERY

A muscle and tissue infection following surgery, well known as a deep incisional surgical site infection (SSI). It affects the soft tissues also surrounding the surgical incision. This infection can extend beyond the superficial skin layers and may originate from an untreated superficial infection or medical devices implanted in your skin. Deep infections necessitate antibiotic therapy, and your doctor may have to fully reopen your incision to drain the infected fluid.

## ORGAN AND BONE INFECTION AFTER SURGERY

An organ and space infection following surgery involves any organ that has been greatly affected or manipulated during the surgical activities. These types of infections can develop from an untreated superficial infection or from bacteria being introduced deep into your body during the surgery.

## INFECTION AFTER SURGERY RISK FACTORS

Infections happen more often in older adults. Health conditions that compromise your system and can increase your risk for an infection include:

**Diabetes.**
**Obesity.**
**Smoking.**
**Prior-skin-infections.**

When to work it out a doctor

If you think that you have an SSI, you ought to contact your doctor right away. Symptoms include:

soreness, pain, and irritation at the location
a fever that spikes at about 100.3°F (38°C) or higher for quite 24 hours
drainage from the location that's cloudy, yellow, tinged with blood, or foul or sweet smelling

## PREVENTING-INFECTIONS

The Centers for Disease Control and Prevention regularly updates recommendations for doctors and hospitals to help prevent Surgical Site Infections (SSIs).You'll also take actions before and after surgery to make an infection less likely to develop.

## BEFORE-SURGERY

Wash with an antiseptic cleanser from the medical practitioner before head to the hospital. Don't shave, as shaving irritates your skin and may introduce infection under your skin. Stop smoking before going for surgery, as smokers develop more infections from trusted Source. Quitting are often very difficult, but it's possible. Speak to a doctor, who can facilitate and develop a quit smoking plan that's good for you.

## AFTER-YOUR-SURGERY

Maintain the sterile dressing that your surgeon applies to your wound for a minimum of 48 hours. Take preventive antibiotics, if prescribed. Make sure you understand how to take care of your wound, asking questions if you would like clarification.

Always wash your hands with soap and water before touching your wound and ask anyone who may assist in your care to try the same. Be proactive within the hospital about your care, listening to how often your wound is being dressed.

# CHAPTER 11

## KITCHEN AND FOOD SAFETY

Preventing gastrointestinal disorder in the kitchen is the ultimate goal of hygiene and food safety standards. No one wants to cause food poisoning, and no one wants to experience it either. So there's a reasonable expectation that food prepared and sold from the kitchen should be done in a manner that prevents food poisoning from happening.

It requires a good understanding of the risks control in the kitchen when it comes to handling foods and other kitchen utensils. This means understanding how bacteria increase and survive also what the risky practices when cooking and displaying foods. Here are 3 quick tips for preventing gastrointestinal disorder in the kitchen:

## 1.CROSS-CONTAMINATION

There are 2 main ways in which germs and bacteria are introduced into the kitchen. Dirty hands

**Raw meats & vegetables**

Hand washing and proper personal hygiene are considered essential for preventing food poisoning. This suggests washing your hands after:

Handling raw foods
Using the rest room
Entering and leaving the kitchen

Separating raw and ready to eat foods is one major way to prevent cross contamination where bacteria can get into foods that shouldn't have. This suggests good storage in the fridges and freezers. Following a color-coding system also helps prevent contamination during the preparation of foods.

## 2. TEMPERATURE CONTROL

Raw meats and vegetables intentionally, naturally have a high bacterial load (high amount of bacteria). Which is why we'd wish to cook meats before we can eat them. Cooking foods to an internal temperature of 75°C (167°F) is considered the safest level to reliably kill harmful bacteria.

Keeping food outside of the critical zone 20 – 45° C (68 – 113° F) eliminates the amount of bacteria that grow.

This pertains to the cooling and defrosting of foods,

as well as the display of foods on a buffet.

Refrigerating foods minimizes the quantity of bacteria that grow.

## 3. CLEANING

A clean and sanitized kitchen ensures that bacteria don't spread within the kitchen. Using suitable cleaning and sanitizing products is vital to eliminate bacteria. this means cleaning crockery, cutlery, cutting boards, equipment and tables on a day to day . Items that inherit contact with food directly need clean-as-you-go, where all other items need daily or weekly cleaning. Rinsing and washing fruits and vegetables is additional element within the control of infections.

Sterilized and clean, and if your caretakers are washing their hands often and wearing gloves when handling your wound.

# CHAPTER 12

# OUT BREAK CONTROL

An outbreak of a disease is defined as two or more cases of a disease related in time and place in excess of normal expectancy.

**Endemic:** Refers to the consistent presence of a disease within a specific geographic area, indicating that it is regularly found in that location.

**Epidemic:** Refers to the occurrence of a group of illnesses in a community or area that is significantly higher than expected, originating from a common or spreadable source.

## TYPES OF OUTBREAKS

Food or waterborne (outbreak team include environmental health officers)

Water (outbreak team include the relevant water company)

For vaccine-preventable diseases, an outbreak team may include vaccination providers to help control the spread. Healthcare-associated infections involve an outbreak team that includes the infection control nurse or doctor. A zoonotic disease is an illness that animals can pass to people. State veterinary service or DEFRA to address the animal-related aspects of the outbreak.

Occupational look backs (outbreak team include occupational health service)

## INVESTIGATING OUTBREAKS

Epidemiological investigations are crucial. you'd like a close knowledge of the suspected disease. as an example , period of time of smallpox is 12 days so one would then concentrate on all contacts with index case 12 days before establish if an outbreak is occurring or has occurred

Define what constitutes a case and choose if the provisional diagnoses fit with this definition.

Act with some speed just just in case the outbreak is genuine.

Treat and isolate the suspected cases.

Start contact tracing.

Initiate microbiological testing, if available

In simple terms you define the event, identify the

cases also collect the data. Then you examine how the disease is being controlled (i.e. identification and treatment of patients). Then, bestir one at preventing the transmission to people and finish up by writing up the experience including lessons learnt so that you can prevent future occurrences and contribute to the epidemiology of outbreaks.

## METHOD FOR OUTBREAK INVESTIGATION

1. Define the outbreak

2. **Define the objectives of outbreak investigation:** Identify source and mode of spread

Interrupt further transmission

Prevent secondary spread

Educate public, healthcare workers involved

Introduce future preventative measures

Prosecute: but need epidemiological and microbiological evidence

## 3. State the steps taken in an epidemic investigation:

Preliminary assessment - is it an outbreak? Confirm numbers, evidence review, form an epidemic or epidemic Control Team, initiate immediate control measures

Develop a case definition and locate instances: considering time, location, individuals, clinical indications, and laboratory findings.

Undertake the descriptive study: collection of data and analysis to urge an epidemic curve you now generate a hypothesis

Undertake an analytical study: case control, use to test the hypothesis - e.g. Cohort study for food outbreaks where the population is well known e.g. reception (attack rate and relative risk ratio) or Case-control study to sample large exposed population odds ratio.

Verify hypothesis using microbiological or environmental tests

## 4. Initiate control measures:

Eradicate source: Treat case, destroy food, and close

shop or eatery

Protect those at risk: hygiene, hand washing and water boiling e.g. stop symptomatic food handlers from working, clean/disinfect premises, recall product immediately.

Prevent recurrence: recommendations, guidelines

5. When communicating with the media, preparing reports, or issuing guidelines, it's important to consider the seriousness of the disease, the discomfort of treatment, and the risk of causing panic within the community.

Additional Factors to give some thought to for Vaccine Preventable Diseases

Outbreak management may include administering follow-up vaccinations to decrease the likelihood of future outbreaks, as seen in cases like measles. This might involve consultants in public health from other public health organization's i.e. screening and immunization leads from PHE/NHSE&I and native public health who will lead on the follow-up actions.

Their involvement will include the following:

Mass communications to high schools and childcare

facilities in the borough, also as primary and secondary healthcare facilities targeted support/resources to the community around the communicable disease and the relevant vaccination liaison with GP surgeries or school aged vaccination providers to rearrange vaccination mop-up for children with incomplete vaccinations plans for catch-up vaccination schemes identification of the gaps within the present vaccination provision and health inequity analysis to inform future commissioning and provision of vaccination services quality improvement of vaccination services.

# CHAPTER 13

# GLOBAL HEALTH SECURITY

A threat from an infectious disease in one region can quickly escalate to a global crisis. Global health security focuses on preventing, detecting, and responding to these infectious threats.

Public health organizations worldwide collaborate to monitor and combat infectious diseases. In the U.S., the Centers for Disease Control and Prevention (CDC) leads efforts to track pathogens, manage outbreaks, and mitigate public health threats. The CDC works closely with national health organizations and the World Health Organization (WHO) to bolster global health.

The CDC emphasized the startling speed at which an infectious disease can spread, moving from a remote village to major cities on different continents in as little as 36 hours. A pathogen threatening one area poses a great risk to all.

Investing in global health security enhances our collective ability to respond to public health threats. Preventing the harmful impacts of diseases and epidemics benefits people around the globe.

## Significant Risks to Global Health Security

Globalization has brought new challenges to health security. Increased interaction between humans and wild animals raises the risk of disease transmission.

Additionally, public health successes have introduced new risks. While antibiotics have saved countless lives, they have also led to drug-resistant pathogens. Smallpox was eradicated globally in the 1970s through vaccination and disease surveillance, yet research labs still hold samples of the virus.

The CDC identifies the top global health security risks today as:

- The outbreak and dissemination of infectious diseases, like the novel coronavirus discovered in 2019
- Increased globalization of trade and travel, which accelerates the spread of diseases
- The emergence of drug-resistant pathogens, such as antibiotic-resistant E. coli
- The potential risk of dangerous pathogens being released intentionally or accidentally

Effective disaster preparation involves understanding these risks Disease surveillance systems allow public health organizations to quickly identify and respond to infectious disease threats.

## Why Disease Surveillance Matters in Public Health.

Disease surveillance is crucial for global health security. It involves tracking and analyzing data related to infectious diseases to monitor public health threats.

Organizations such as the CDC and WHO gather and analyze data on disease outbreaks and their patterns of spread. The CDC's Division of High-Consequence Pathogens and Pathology (DHCPP) focuses on the most contagious and deadly pathogens, while the WHO's Health Emergencies Program continuously monitors high-threat diseases. Data from these surveillance systems provide early warnings about potential public health threats.

Disease surveillance offers several benefits to public health organizations, including tracking dangerous infectious diseases, limiting pathogen spread, and improving health outcomes.

*George Leo*

## Tracking Dangerous Pathogens

Surveillance systems track harmful pathogens to prevent them from developing into epidemics. The DHCPP in the U.S. These systems use networks to monitor diseases like anthrax, rabies, hantavirus, and others. In collaboration with the WHO and other global public health organizations, the DHCPP works to mitigate the impact of outbreaks.

In addition to monitoring known pathogens, disease surveillance organizations like the DHCPP identify new infectious diseases. They test unknown agents to assess potential threats, enabling early detection efforts such as the rapid sequencing of COVID-19, which facilitated the accelerated development of a vaccine.

## Prevention of Disease Spread

By detecting outbreaks early, disease surveillance systems play a key role in preventing and controlling the spread of diseases. These systems study how diseases spread to handle and prevent transmission.

Public health organizations employ several techniques to prevent disease spread. They first identify the pathogen causing the outbreak, then trace its source, and finally monitor disease transmission to implement prevention strategies or recommend other interventions.

## Improving Public Health Outcomes

The ultimate goal of disease surveillance is to enhance public health outcomes. Early warning systems help contain disease spread and minimize the impact of infectious diseases.

In addition to tracking pathogens and limiting disease spread, public health surveillance aids policymakers. Organizations can better plan, set priorities, and improve health outcomes based on surveillance data.

These organizations also evaluate how effective various public health interventions are. By analyzing and comparing strategies, they determine which interventions have the greatest impact on public health.

## The Pillars of Global Health Security

Promoting global health requires a collaborative response. While early detection can pinpoint outbreaks, these efforts may fail without a robust response system. Similarly, a strong healthcare infrastructure is essential for successful emergency response.

## Preventing Global Health Risks

Shielding global well-being commences with thwarting the proliferation of pathogens. This crucial task involves not only forestalling the genesis of harmful pathogens but also averting the unleashing of contained infectious ailments. In times of outbreaks, prevention emerges as a potent weapon in the arsenal of public health, solidifying its status as a cornerstone of global health security.

## Detecting Impending Threats

Vigilance against diseases underscores the importance of surveillance systems dedicated to monitoring public health hazards. Each nation employs diverse methodologies and institutions to discern the propagation of pathogens. Surveillance, laboratory analysis, and robust reporting mechanisms stand pivotal in this detection process. Achieving global health necessitates a concerted endeavor by national public health bodies, entailing the sharing of information to safeguard global well-being.

## Responding to Emergencies

Beyond prevention and detection, swift response

remains pivotal in fortifying global health. Effective communication and coordination facilitate the mobilization of resources during public health crises. This pillar encompasses readiness for emergencies, meticulous planning for disaster responses, and effective dissemination of critical information.

## Strengthening Health Infrastructure

The resilience of national health infrastructures plays a pivotal role in ensuring public health security globally. Throughout the COVID-19 pandemic, numerous health systems grappled with surges in healthcare demand and shortages of essential medical resources. Robust health systems serve to mitigate the risks posed by public health crises.

## Upholding International Standards

The foundation of global health security rests upon the adherence of nations to international norms governing disease surveillance and public health promotion. This pillar encompasses compliance with standards in public health financing and emergency protocols.

## Assessing Unique Risks

Diverse nations confront distinct risk landscapes concerning public health, spanning vulnerabilities to biological threats, political instabilities, and infrastructural deficiencies. This pillar endeavors to address the multifaceted infectious disease and health risks prevalent across nations.

The Global Health Security Index: A Pillar of Preparedness

The Global Health Security Index establishes benchmarks for health security, evaluating the preparedness of 195 nations. Spearheaded by the Nuclear Threat Initiative (NTI) and the Johns Hopkins Center for Health Security (Johns Hopkins CHS), the GHS Index commenced in October 2019.

Utilizing the six pillars of global health security, the GHS Index consistently gauges public health capabilities. In 2021, the Index disaggregated these six categories into 37 indicators and 171 inquiries, prioritizing preparedness, environmental hazards, adherence to global public health standards, and the robustness of national health systems.

This data spotlight health security shortcomings at

the national level, enabling countries to allocate resources towards preempting future outbreaks. For instance, public health entities and governmental bodies can utilize the GHS Index to pinpoint areas necessitating further investment and strategic planning.

The GHS Index intends to undertake assessments biennially or triennially to monitor emergency preparedness, fostering a continuous pursuit of global health security.

# CONCLUSION

Control and Prevention of Infectious Diseases stands as a pillar of hope and knowledge in the ongoing battle against infectious diseases. It is a testament to human resilience and the power of collective effort in combating these relentless foes. Through the pages of this book, we have witnessed the devastating impact of infectious diseases on individuals, families, and communities, but we have also seen the triumphs of science, medicine, and public health in controlling and preventing their spread.

This book serves as a reminder of the importance of vigilance and preparedness in the face of emerging infectious threats. It emphasizes the critical role of education, research, and global cooperation in addressing these challenges.

*George Leo*

As we navigate the complexities of our modern world, Control and Prevention of Infectious Diseases serves as a guidepost, offering insights and strategies to protect ourselves and future generations from the ravages of infectious diseases.

www.ingramcontent.com/pod-product-compliance
Lightning Source LLC
Chambersburg PA
CBHW070426240526
45472CB00020B/1461